THE TRUTH ABOUT HAIR LOSS

WHAT YOU NEED TO KNOW ABOUT YOUR
HAIR, TREATMENT, AND PREVENTION

ROBERT RICHARD

CONTENTS

FOREWORD

"I have been utilizing Robert's techniques and after 2 weeks I have seen fuzz on my bald spots, already! I can't thank the author enough for this book." - Dustin Robinson

"I've been doing this for just under two months and my frontal hairline is coming back." - Timothy Walker

"I was skeptical at first but it was easy to do, and I had nothing to lose. I just can't believe I'm getting results. My wife loves touching my hair again." - Anthony Ferrer

"I was frustrated with my hair loss and then I got this title; all I can say is 'WOW'" - Jeremiah Tobias

ACKNOWLEDGEMENTS

I'd like to thank many people on my road to getting my hair back, because without their hard years of research I wouldn't have this thick mane of hair that I do now. I also wouldn't be able to have helped so many people in the process, either. So; firstly, I'd like to thank the people at http://www.hairloss-research.org/ because their research is top notch and they have helped 1000s of people with their hair loss issues, along with their scientific research on multiple products. I'd also like to thank Dr. Stephen T. Chang for his devotion into putting many years of hard work into his many titles that gave great insight into the system of the human body as a whole. I can't tell you enough about how this was of great support in my own hair loss journey. And, lastly, my friends, my family and my wonderful wife who supported my bald head for so long, and gave me the confidence to write this title! Thank you all.

PREFACE

We are living in the age of ignorance; a world of fake news, misinformation, and lies. It is a truly corporate dictatorship. I see this to be most prevalent in the healthcare system. It's not about helping and healing anymore; it's all about those dollar signs. They want to control the symptom, NOT cure it, and they charge you every step of the way for the rest of your life.

It only takes a little researching into the (not so distant) past to see how ignorant and "sheepworthy" people are. One example we all can relate to is cigarettes. Those corporations spent millions and millions promoting the fact that they had no adverse health effects, but now it's just common knowledge that those things are just "cancer wrapped up in a stick." Or how about this, I bet you didn't know it… in the 30s right up until the mid 50s, they used to (commonly) use radioactive ingredients in everyday household items! This included skin care products for women, radioactive chocolate bars, cigarettes (of course), watches, and even toothpaste! Imagine that, putting a generation-destroying substance in your body on a daily basis. And, more recently, we were told that after a brain cell dies it doesn't regenerate. The BS that they used to promote! Wow, what a load of crap. It makes me really frustrated and angry. I am a truth seeker, just so you know, right from the get-go.

So, while we're on the topic of greedy sociopathic corporations, let's talk about those strands of hair on your head that are falling out, and the only "medicine" doctors say that can do anything to fix it. The ones these doctors "or Big Pharma drug dealers" (as I call them) keep telling you to take. The ones that literally kill you from the inside out, cost an arm and a leg, and do little to nothing at all. Oh, and once you stop taking them what little you gained falls out anyway! Ugh...

OR, we can talk about proven ways that will cost you next-to-nothing! Yes, the wonderful ideas and answers that WILL benefit your health, without making you sick. And, with REAL results which are permanent. It's a pretty obvious choice, right? I want you to keep your hard-earned money in your pocket, and I want you to take your money out of those doctors/so-called experts' pockets... but most of all I want to help you get your hair back; all of it! Yes, hairline and all, with none of this 'artificial-thickening it up BS' that's so prevalent in the marketplace these days.

So, in this title you will learn the main cause of male pattern baldness in detail, including the whys and the hows of it all. Additionally, I will also explain how to prevent and reverse it naturally, healthily, and without spending hours of your time and money on utter BS. So, with that; let's begin!

MY HAIR LOSS STORY

Hi, my name is Robert Richard. When I was in my 20s I first started noticing my hair loss in the prime of my life; when I was single and working full-time. Basically, at the time, I would get up in the morning each day, and triple-check the pillowcase for hair. It was horrible. Every single day... the first thing I thought about was my hair!

I would religiously wash my hair with some kind of "grow your hair back" kind of shampoo (I think I had a half a cupboard full of them at one point in time).

I tried every brand on the market and "enhanced" formulations that were dedicated to reverse the hair loss and get me my hair back. I think I was close to paranoid. Hoping no more would fall out, and squinting my eyes in the mirror to check for more growth. It was pure craziness, really.

Anyway, at the worst point of it all, I began losing multiple hairs every day when I washed it with shampoos that were supposed to "magically" help it grow back... somehow. And when it was at its absolute worst, I lost as many as 200 hairs in a single wash! I had a hair catcher in the bottom of my shower, believe it or not. This was something that put me into a state of paranoia!

Each day, I continued on this path of hope. Hoping that (somehow) everything would become normal again, and that I wouldn't be that guy who was losing hair and slowly balding. I had quite-literally become obsessed by this state of anxious behaviour, one that sent me into a whirlwind of "No, not today, please." Pretty embarrassing, I know, but that's how much it affected my life, and I'm sure I'm not the only one who has been affected in this way.

It was like the movie, *Groundhog Day*, every day I would immediately think about my hair, over and over again in a constant state of "dejavu."

I would then take my shower, after checking my pillow and counting hairs, and then I would count the ones caught in the drain catcher, too. Basically, I found myself living my life like the problem had "overtaken" me. And, of course, it had.

After I figured everything out, which took some months of research, I fixed my problem and the anxiety that drove me went away. Thank goodness. I could even concentrate and sleep much easier.

As the change occurred, I felt like a new man; renewed in a way, like I was somehow getting my whole life back again. And this was pivotal for me.

Finally... Success Came...

After implementing my knowledge and using trial and error for the techniques, I worked out that I really was able reverse my hair loss. And, I learned that; if I kept utilizing the techniques, I would be able to regrow and restore my hair growth completely, and naturally.

Over time, the recovery of my hair was major, and as a result, today I enjoy a bountiful head of hair, again. My stress and anxiety has completely subsided, too.

It's true; hair loss is a horrible condition to have. When it strikes, it just seems to keep getting worse and worse, to the point where you can lose hope altogether, which is not good.

After trying loads of things, I needed to have a completely natural solution. I want to tell you – hair loss is reversible, for men and women, yes; both sexes. By applying these techniques I used, you can keep the hair you still have and regrow the hair you've lost. So, let's go, I have so much information to share with you! I can't wait to disclose absolutely everything!! Thanks for being here with me. It's your lucky day...

1

THE RELATIONSHIP BETWEEN HAIR LOSS & SCALP BLOOD CIRCULATION

So most men (by age 50) suffer from a heavy-type of hair loss which is called *Androgenic Alopecia Areata* or "male pattern baldness." But, it's also the case that some men begin losing hair in their early 20s. Sometimes women do too. For them, though, it is usually-always stress or illness related. The reasons behind the problem for males can vary greatly. Hair loss can be causational, and driven by hormonal changes in the male body, it can occur from excessive stress, as a side effect of certain medications, or even because of genetics.

In recent times, "Big Pharma" and mainstream media only gave the globe a few "available" solutions regarding the problem. Two of the major ones were *hair transplantation* and *prescription medications*.

But let's get this clear about something first before we begin, you might say to me, "But Robert, my friend eats this, my friends use this shampoo, and their hair is perfectly fine... how can you say it's damaging to mine or is a cause for hair loss?"

Unfortunately, we're not all the same, and that's a plain and simple fact of life. Some people have more DHT receptors in the scalp and accumulate it higher than others, and some people have less circulation than others do. You will understand more about these factors soon. Let's be totally clear here. We are all UNIQUE; genetically, physically, and individually. Many physical traits are the end result of a complex interjection between an individual's genes and the environment that surrounds them. But male pattern baldness appears to be extremely dependent on genetic gearing. Female pattern baldness is even more distinctive, and appears to be caused by other factors.

"If you look at identical twins — who share 100 percent of their genes — typically, they have a very similar pattern of hair loss," states Markus Nöthen, a professional geneticist at the University of Bonn, Germany.

He learned that between 79 and 81 percent of baldness was due to genetics and genes of the individual in the case of men.

So anyway when comes to the subject of the relationship between hair loss & scalp blood circulation the topic is not always spoken about when hair loss is "covered," pardon the pun. But, in truth, it's extremely important to understand. We'll talk about the fundamental aspects that are pivotal to getting acquainted with this section of the knowledge base.

Actually, I bought several pills, lotions, and shampoos in my journey, and I came to the conclusion that none of these were right for me. None. They didn't work and I felt at a loss to understand why. I was frustrated, disappointed, and really sick and tired of buying things that didn't help me in any way, shape or form.

In fact, once I started on my path to finding out about hair loss, I read every article, book, and medical title I could follow. I just had to know how I could change my "lot" in life. I didn't want to be "the bald guy," not in my 20s, anyway. And, if possible, not in my old age, either.

I was particularly interested in the information I read concerning blood circulation in general. This made real sense to me.

I found out some interesting facts about circulation with regard to hair growth and hair loss; let's have a look at some of them now.

Hair loss can be due to:

- The decrease in the micro blood circulation on the top part of the head;
- The blood circulation issue can occur in the frontal, temporal, vertex and occipital zones of the head;
- When blood circulation is lessened in these areas, the hair follicles can't achieve enough blood flow necessary to maintain healthy growth;
- Blood flow is always necessary for good hair growth and loss prevention, overall;
- From there (no proper circulation) the follicles remain in an inactive state, causing them to become dormant

Following on from these points, the hair follicles that remain inactive now finish their life cycle and fall out. And I definitely knew what this was like. I didn't like it at all. And also, there can be certain areas where this becomes obvious, and that is where the term "balding" springs from. This issue is usually the main cause of hair loss or "balding" in people who have trouble with this issue. This is true in 80 to 90 percent of cases.

The peripheral (or outer) blood circulation is responsible for giving oxygen and other nutrients to the hair follicles. This is necessary to sustain a constant supply of much-needed constituents for the hair growth to continue after the old follicle has fallen out. Amino acids, vitamins, minerals, and proteins are distributed via the bloodstream. These variables can be changed via the foods and drinks we consume, and any supplements we take, as well. There is, therefore, a direct connection to food consumption and hair growth or loss, from person to person, with regard to blood flow success. It's also true that the oxygenation of the blood will occur more healthily, and when an individual has a healthy diet, overall. This makes a huge difference in the way our hair reacts or performs, too. There is a definite signalling link between hair health and diet, which then becomes a necessity for hair loss and the prevention of loss in the long-term, for the individual in question. We will look at this a little later in the title. So, stay tuned for that.

Let's stay on track. Actually, in order to stimulate blood vessels, the focus must be on the top area of the scalp. The products that I used, and there were multiple, didn't do this. And, it was the reason for failure and my devastation, time and time again.

What can cause hair loss? So far, I knew that stress and heredity could be issues, as well as nutrition, which we'll discuss soon. But what else? I needed to know... everything. I found out a little more information about stress, and that muscle tenseness occurred when individuals were stressed. I also learned that certain chemicals produced while in this state could affect the follicles at the base, therefore, cutting off the blood supply. Additionally, stress can increase the oils on the scalp, resulting in an "oily scalp." This then leads to suffocation of the capillary follicles.

After research from multiple sources, I came to a realization about hair loss. Why was it that no one ever seemed to lose hair above their ears, or on the back of their lower neck? Everywhere else seemed to be a place for baldness, and I looked at many scales and images as I researched this fact, and noticed that there was a definite connection. But, it took me a while longer to "click" on the areas I was still puzzled about. I was mystified about my questions regarding hair loss areas, and I wanted a scientific and valid explanation to tell me why it was so.

After a time, I stumbled onto something I found extremely enlightening. When an individual partook in physical exercise, the body would react with a vasodilation of the blood cells. Opening them up, so the blood flow could increase to the muscular tissues. The diameter of the blood capillaries becomes increased, and this allows for blood to circulate far more easily. And this fact was like finding gold for me, the knowledge kind. I already realized that my diet was an important factor, and now I also realized that blood flow could also be affected by physical exercise, as well.

I kept going, and I learned more valuable information. And then it dawned on me as I looked in the mirror and I saw muscles on my temples moving as I was shaving!

You've guessed it already, haven't you?

There are some areas that get more exercise than others! When you eat and talk, these muscles are exercised in certain places in the head, more specifically, the temporal and auricular muscles. Yes, the ones in the mid-section of the head and behind the ears.

It's true, it's not that well-known, but we have muscles on the top of the head too (the frontal-occipital and the galea, which joins these facets together) in this section. But how could I activate the blood vessels in the areas of my scalp that weren't being exercised, voluntarily? This was my challenge over the next month or so. I looked everywhere, searching for answers, because, in reality, that's all I really needed to do. I wanted to know why the circulation wasn't occurring in the top and mid-sections of people's heads. And it wasn't just due to a lack of physical movement there, or so I found out. Actually, the extremities of the body naturally don't get as much blood flow, because the body needs this more definitively for the organs, like the heart and lungs. These are geared toward survival, and so, it is a fact that the outer extremities lack blood flow, compared to the other areas which are closer to the vital organs.

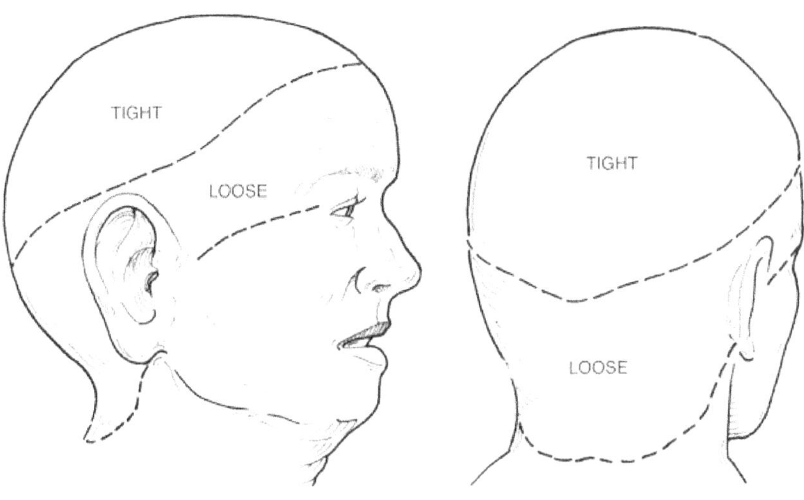

During the time I was searching, I came up without many more answers. And, I was getting more and more frustrated, knowing that all I really needed to do was increase blood flow to the area that my hair follicles had been falling out, and to lower stress and eat well, nutritionally.

So, I kept delving and diving into more and more information. I spent hours and hours looking for scientific incorporations, and anything else that might help my cause. Statistically, it seemed the odds were against me. And... even celebrities and movie stars who had money still wore toupees. So, obviously, they didn't even have any answers. Now I became more disheartened, thinking that I was stuck with my hair loss, and that I would eventually go bald. And, there would be no product that would work, especially if it was stress reduction, nutrition, and physical exercise that needed to be in play. What I really needed was a great, proven methodology or a system that worked hands-down. I really didn't want to go bald in my 20's. It just wasn't something that I could contend with, either emotionally or socially. So far, I already knew that stress reduction, nutrition, and physical exercise in certain areas (that I hadn't found yet) were necessary. I needed to keep going. And I did, with more passion and fervor than I ever thought was possible. Let's continue, shall we?

2

DHT THE HORMONAL DESTROYER FOR HAIR

THIS SUBJECT WILL ALLOW US TO UNDERSTAND A BIT MORE about DHT, the altered form of testosterone. It has been scientifically proven that this hormone is detrimental in the hair loss arena. In fact, studies show that this hormone (when seen in elevated levels) led to hair loss in participants who were scientifically studied, in multiple research groups.

The studies showed that DHT:

1. Makes hair finer

2. Makes hair weaker

3. Miniaturizes hair through a combination of the problems mentioned in both (1.) and (2.)

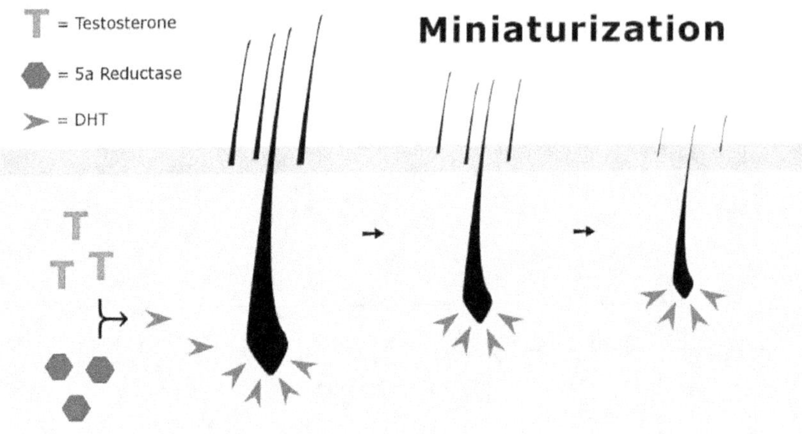

This widely unknown cause for hair loss is why so many hair products don't work. And, now we know 4 major reasons for the cause of hair loss, so far:

1. Stress (general stress can cause muscle tension and oily scalp issues)

2. Nutrition deficiencies (including foods that need to be consumed and avoided)

3. Lack of physical exercise in certain areas pertaining to the muscles in the head

4. Increases in the DHT hormone

So, how is testosterone transformed into DHT, the "enemy" chemical that causes hair loss? And is it really the enemy? Let's see...

Testosterone is converted by an enzyme (called 5-alpha reductase) which changes the form of it into DHT. There are two types that are produced, the first occurs in the sebaceous glands which are located in the oiliest part of the follicle, and the second occurs inside the follicle itself. In time, DHT keeps being produced which makes the hair follicle go into its inactive state; called dormancy. Eventually, the hair becomes finer, weaker, and then miniaturizes before it falls out, altogether.

Over the course of history, DHT has been dubbed "an enemy" or "the devil hormone" because of its effects on hair loss, overall. But, in actual fact, the male body needs DHT, very-much so. It is responsible for the development and formation of the male sexual characteristics on the whole. It is, quite literally, the hormone needed to transmute a boy into a man, and sustain that change, right from adolescence and into adulthood. Without DHT the male body can behave very strangely.

Unfortunately, many products have surfaced on the current market. These are ones which have been specifically made to lessen and control DHT formation and production within the body. And unfortunately, this can have detrimental effects on a man and his functioning, overall. The main point I am trying to make here is that; lessening DHT is absolutely necessary. But, this is **only true** for the scalp area, and **not the entire body**, as a whole entity.

Some of the detrimental effects can include:

• Loss of appetite for sex

• Impotency (in men)

• Erectile dysfunction (in men)

• Female breast development (in men)

Drugs like Propecia (finasteride) have had shocking long-term effects on men, who need to continue the treatment at a cost of over $700 per year, because of the impermanence of its functioning methodology. This means that; for hair loss to be impeded, an individual would need this ongoing treatment for the rest of their lifetime and, at the detriment of their health both now and in the long-term. Discontinuing the use of products like Propecia will create the issue again. The need for pills like this is not suggested.

It was a natural way that I was looking for. I knew that I didn't want to become impotent, or have erectile dysfunction, either. No thanks. The other harrowing problems were large breast formation and a low sexual appetite. These conditions definitely weren't for me, either. I needed a way to keep my testosterone from changing into DHT, but in the scalp only, if this was even possible at all.

I kept searching, and then I stumbled upon some research that made me get excited. The study found that it was possible to convert DHT back into testosterone via the use of voluntary muscles! In fact, it was possible to reactivate the parts of my scalp that had dying hair roots, due to the production of DHT, and in the areas that were being affected. It was like a bonanza of much needed and hoped-for knowledge. This information can be sourced from Wikipedia when you look up "Dihydrotestosterone" (the long name for DHT). It was there (and via a few other sources) that I learned that there was an enzyme that can reconvert DHT back into testosterone. It is called "3-alpha hydroxysteroid dehydrogenase." This enzyme is not detrimental to hair growth, so it might be the answer I'd longed for. I felt so excited about what I found.

I kept reading and found out even more. Dr. Bryan J. Freund D.D.S., M.D. (Ontario, Canada) incorporated a scientific study that was based upon the formation of DHT. It surmised the need for excellent blood circulation and the need for proper vasodilation of the capillaries as major factors for success, overall. The study was called "Treatment of Male Pattern Baldness with Botulinum Toxin."

The findings suggested that:

1. Conversion from testosterone to DHT was favored in low oxygen environments at a cellular level.

2. DHT, when given more oxygenation, changed itself into another hormone, one that was not associated with hair loss.

3. Areas above the neck and ears are prone to oxygenation because they are moved regularly, during jaw movement in eating, talking, or facial expression changes. This prevents both the production and the accumulation of the hormone known as DHT.

4. The areas prone to less oxygenation aren't physically moved, leading to a lessened amount of blood flow to those areas, thus increasing the DHT production there, and leading to thinning, and eventual hair loss, over time.

5. Overproduction of DHT can also irritate the sebaceous glands to action and create sebum, which is rich in DHT hormone, signaling even more hair loss to occur.

Two major factors are necessary for hair loss to stop:

1. Oxygenation is necessary

2. Circulation is required to stop DHT formation that needs oxygen

I felt wonderful as I found myself understanding why men and women went bald. I was getting closer to something. But who else knew about this? And how could this be fixed?

I had to find someone who understood this; because I was young and at my peak. I read more, and even though I knew plenty already, I still needed to understand how it affected women. Women had these issues too, and it must be devastating for them, considering that social values are geared to looking great, in this extremely "looks mean everything" time that we now live in. Self-esteem could be really low for men who had hair loss issues, but women... wow, that could be just as gruelling, if not more daunting for them. Anyway, I found out that women, when stressed, produce more testosterone, and then, the oxygenation issue easily comes into play, in the same way it does for men.

So, now, this issue was big... I realized that it was affecting so many. And people all around the entire globe. Demographics didn't matter, but stress, nutrition, physical exercise, oxygenation, and circulation mattered... A LOT. But I had tried nearly every product around, and obviously, no one company knew about this yet, or did they? I needed to find out. I would eventually, because I was on the precipice of fixing my issue.

3

TREAT & RESOLVE SCALP CONDITIONS WITH THESE GREAT TIPS

LET'S TAKE A LOOK AT THE SEBACEOUS GLANDS. I RESEARCHED these because they also contain DHT in the sebum. The sebaceous glands sit at the base of the follicle and must maintain the right amount of sebum for greater functioning. Sebum is composed of fat, keratin, dead skin cells, and a high concentration of the hormone DHT. With the important role of hydration and protection, sebum is necessary for healthy hair to be maintained. Too much is not good, nor is too little. Balancing its production is, therefore, important to prevent conditions like dandruff or dermatitis.

Supplements to help with conditions would need to include: magnesium, copper, iron, selenium, zinc, sulfur, and vitamins A, B (from the biotin group), C, and E. It's often the case that issues begin with certain skin irritations or dandruff. That's how you know that there is an overproduction or an underproduction of sebum.

The skin cells on the surface of the skin are continually replaced, and if the overproduction or underproduction occurs, it can put the skin in that area into a troublesome pattern. An accelerated replacement of cells can occur with increased sebum production. The skin will try to keep up and then begins shedding cells before they reach full growth. The surface cells (made up of fat and dead cells) impede circulation, and this can suffocate and impede hair roots, leading to issues that can create untoward symptoms and limit hair cell growth in both the short and long-term. This condition is known as seborrhea.

The importance of regulating sebum is paramount because it contains DHT, which we already know creates hair loss, and eventually (at its worst) can cause balding in both men and women. The two types of seborrhea are "fatty" and "dry." The fatty seborrhea condition is comprised by these constituents of the scalp: being scaly, itchy, oily, and having white/yellowish flakes that are obvious on the scalp. The dry seborrhea condition is comprised of dry, itchy flakes, with white corneal cells falling off that are known as dandruff.

There are 3 Major Causes of Seborrhea:

1. **Adolescent** - This promotes more sebum via increased hormonal production during this time of life.

2. **Nutritional** - Bad diet with an excess of fried or fatty foods, and the blood becomes full of excess fat, irritating the glands which then produce more sebum. Cutting out simple carbs, avoiding excess red meat consumption, sugars, dairy, and wheat is necessary. Replace these with complex carbs including brown rice, pasta, vegetables, white meat, seafood, soy, and beans.

3. **Nervous** - Caused primarily by high levels of stress, thus, resulting in muscle tension and the lack of blood flow to certain areas,

allowing DHT production to be rife, due to less oxygenation in those areas.

Alleviate Seborrhea by:

- Don't scratch or itch the scalp because it irritates the sebaceous glands that produce more sebum
- Cutting the hair shorter can help increase its tonicity, and also reduces the increase and stagnation of sebum, improving the general health of the scalp
- The right shampoo is paramount, for PH incorporation that is fitting to the individual

The right shampoo is paramount. Using a good cleanser is important. Many people (1 in 5) are affected by shampoos that are too aggressive in nature. When talking about shampoo, it's important we understand that the PH or alkalinity/acidity factor is vitally important. The skin reacts best to organic and natural products. We need to use shampoos without coloring agents or additives, which will help with the regulation of sebum and block DHT.

There are 3 types of hair; oily, dry and normal hair. As an example, oily hair is usually denoted by a person who also has oily skin, in general. It gets dirtier more often and needs to be constantly washed. The recommended shampoo for this type of hair is made up of factors that mean the shampoo is organic, natural, and derived from plant-based constituents. It should not contain parabens, foaming agents, sulfates, SLS, chemical agents, and/or SLES. These remove and compromise the hair follicles. Regular use of a great shampoo will alleviate dandruff and itching. A great shampoo will also support the sebum production, which is vitally important for issues of hair loss.

Dry hair is denoted by the hydration of skin being off balance.

Prolonged use of aggressive shampoo is harmful. Itching can be annoying. Here, we need a delicate product that rehydrates the scalp.

Normal hair is really balanced. So, it just needs a great shampoo with natural, organic, and balanced constituents to support the growth.

Let's take a look at shampoos. These are important if itching, dandruff, and/or irritation are a problem. Treating these conditions is paramount, because these conditions can signify a presence of micro-organisms that feed on the sebum. They are scientifically called *pityrosporum ovale* and can live on the scalp, impeding your hair, and are a type of fungus. If these conditions are not dealt with, these micro-organisms can multiply and change the sebum they consume into acid fats, which irritates the sebaceous glands on a detrimental level. The scalp sheds even more, leading to damaged scalp and hair.

I'll have a chapter later on with recipes on some natural shampoos you can make all natural but really you can use baking soda. baking soda, a substance easy to find in the grocery store. Add one tablespoon to a cup of hot water and stir in well. Place this mixture into a clean container. Using a well-washed old shampoo container works well. This is completely natural and works extremely well to alleviate conditions of the scalp associated with dermatitis or dandruff issues. In the shower, rub it on the scalp, and leave it on for about 4 minutes. It won't strip your hair of vital nutrients. Make sure you rinse your hair thoroughly.

If you have dry hair, add a little less baking soda to your mixture, for oily hair you can add a little more. Trial and error might be necessary for your unique hair type. Once you find a great match, you can use it whenever a condition begins to plague you. This is a cheap way to fix the problem, and it works extremely well. Some people use it every day and others use it as an anti-dandruff shampoo twice a week. Most people find that it works wonders on their hair. In unusual cases, it might irritate skin in some instances. Do a test on a part of the scalp, first. You might need to use it for a fortnight to see results regarding the issue of dandruff. It has a PH of around 9. As an addition, a great natural conditioning product can be utilized by mixing *natural apple cider vinegar* and mixing this with *water*.

Personally, I avoided using shampoo - using only water and scrubbing to clean my hair (both to reduce sebum production and to avoid potentially hormone-disrupting chemicals being placed on my scalp). I used a boar bristle brush after my hair was dry to give it that clean and conditioned look, without poisoning my hair.

I wanted to mention the reason why I don't need to use damaging conditioners, and why my boar bristle brush is the perfect solution because it very overlooked item in your arsenal.

Since the 1800s, boar bristle brushes have been used to create shiny-looking, vital hair without the use of products. Boar bristle brushes were also seen on dressing tables during the first part of the 20th century as a commonplace regularity. Stars like Lauren Bacall, Rita Hayworth, Katherine Hepburn, and other magnetizing movie greats were able to obtain their pivotal, shiny hairstyles by incorporating the use of this brushing into their regime.

The benefits of Boar bristle include:

1. **Naturally Conditions the Hair**

This type of brushing is a conditioning treatment. While it does boast some great styling elements, it was originally designed to improve the texture and shine of hair before products even existed. The amazing structure of the brush carries sebum, which is the oil produced by the scalp, and right from the scalp to the end of the hair shaft. It works by coating each strand of hair with a very small amount of sebum, therefore, (quite literally) adding lustrous shine.

2. **Improves the Hair's Texture**

It seems to help positively with regard to the texture of hair as well. The design and implication allows the hair to look great. If you have straight hair it will add volume and shine that bounces. If you have curly hair it will slightly loosen the curl and condition it.

3. Reduces Frizziness

Sebum is the most effective anti-frizz serum. By using the brush to lubricate each hair with sebum, you'll notice a big reduction in the frizz factor!

4. Stimulates the Scalp

The brushing incorporates a meditative and relaxing feeling, overall. The brush feels wonderful on the scalp and stimulates the right blood flow to the hair follicles, which can also enhance hair growth, long-term.

5. Reduces the Need for Products

As your hair becomes shinier, more vibrant, and "beams out" from great health, it will feel softer and more conditioned with continued daily brushing, so that means you'll no longer need to use products that take away the vitality and health of your hair.

6. Reduces the Frequency of Needing to Wash Your Hair

A boar bristle brush can help you maintain healthy and clean hair. It also prevents the oil buildup on the scalp, which weighs hair down and makes it look oily. You may find that you can reduce the frequency of hair washing to every two, three, four, or even five days at a time. Wow, what an amazing tool.

4

DON'T USE FDA-APPROVED DRUGS
FOR HAIR LOSS

THERE IS MUCH EVIDENCE TO SHOW US THAT THERE ARE MANY corporations and marketing companies who want you to believe there is little that men and women can do to stop them from losing their hair. In fact, they try and promote only a limited amount of pharmacological medications which are available at great risk to customers.

There are two current medications: Propecia and Rogaine – both approved by the U.S. Federal Drug Administration (FDA) for the tackling of hair loss. They have been studied and clinically proven to show an element of some effectiveness, but with a cost to health as I explained earlier.

It is true that these medications for hair loss can slow further thinning of hair and support increased coverage of the scalp by promoting new hair growth and enlarging the existing hairs. However, these have to be taken continuously, and once a medication is stopped, any hair which has grown back will gradually be lost again, and, within 12 months you could find the scalp is back as it was before you started.

Propecia (finasteride) and Rogaine (minoxidil) work entirely differently in their applications. Propecia is a pill you take once per day, while Rogaine is a fluid which you apply to the scalp twice per day. Propecia and Rogaine have not been proven to restore hair in the frontal areas, because they don't target all of the causes necessary for permanent results.

Propecia Disadvantages

- Propecia doesn't cure hair loss, and it will only work over the long-term if you continue using it. If you stop taking Propecia, you will more-than-likely lose any hair growth you've gained within 12 months of stopping treatment.
- Propecia is not approved or recommended for use by women, at all.
- Sexual side effects, such as decreased sexual desire, and struggling to achieve erections.
- Endless treatment with Propecia will work out expensive and require lifetime usage.
- Female-looking breasts can be grown due to the lessened DHT hormone throughout the whole body, not just the scalp.

Rogaine Disadvantages

- Rogaine doesn't cure hair loss, and it will only work over the long-term if you continue using it. If you stop taking

Rogaine, you will more-than-likely lose any hair growth you've gained.

- Limited effectiveness. Rogaine treatment won't work for everybody with thinning hair. Especially inherited pattern hair loss. It is far less efficient for any hair loss at the hairline than it is on the top of the head. It is less useful on larger sized bald spots than smaller ones.
- Might not help men with severe balding at all.
- Some men purely don't like putting lotion on their scalp.
- It has a high cost, and it is not covered by health insurance schemes because it falls under a cosmetic application.

As you can see, these two methods are a real waste of your money and can come with a heftier price to more than just your wallet. The health risks are far from worth it, especially when there might be little to no results at all! Ghastly... So now, let's expand on the nutritional causes of hair loss, and how we can correct these in ways that won't poison us, or waste our precious time and money.

Hair Transplantation

This technique is a surgical procedure that is rather expensive, very painful, and also very dangerous. A positive result is not guaranteed. I would never suggest this method to anyone. The average cost of hair transplantation is around $8000, depending upon your country and location. Please know that some surgeons are not even qualified or they may have a lack of experience, altogether. DO NOT risk your health for this. Actually, you have a great risk of losing all of your healthy hair, because of the shock created by surgery. Additionally, you may obtain awful scars, excessive stress, and lose self-confidence from the trauma of it not working.

5

THE CAUSES OF ANXIETY
HAIR LOSS

WHEN IT COMES TO STRESS AND ANXIETY, BOTH WESTERN AND eastern philosophies on healing both agree. This detrimental damage can wreak havoc on the body. So, in this chapter I will discuss its effects on hair, and how to resolve any stress or anxiety as much as possible.

Hair loss is never just the only symptom of anxiety, and it is also very rare for your hair loss to occur if your anxiety levels aren't severe.

The critical issues between anxiety and an individual's hair loss are stress. In a way, anxiety is long-term, and made up of continuing stress. While in theory, these being two separate conditions, the reality is, anyone who is dealing with anxiety is placing themselves under severe physical and mental pressure all of the time.

Now it's time to not only reduce your stress and anxiety but also increase the circulation and blood to your scalp at the same time! How you might ask? A sauna and steams rooms are the best answers.

Clears the Skin:

Steam helps clear skin impurities and can actually be used to treat acne. It can also help to improve circulation all over the body, which gives skin a healthy glow making you look and feel great, too.

Relieving Tension:

The heat from the sauna will soothe your nerve endings and also relax your muscles. A lesser well-known benefit of both saunas and steam rooms is that they minimize joint pain, and also act in minimizing the pains from headaches, due to their high-heat environments.

If you have regular access to a steam room or a sauna; then that's excellent. If not, you can soak in a bathtub with the temperature higher than your body's, for 10 minutes. Set a timer. DO NOT perspire for more than 10 minutes or you will lose too much nutrition from the nutrients which escape (in the liquid being eliminated) through the pores.

Removes Toxins:

The heat from sauna and steam rooms makes your body sweat.

Sweating relieves the body of waste products, and it is known that sitting in a sauna or steam room for around twenty minutes can rid the body of the day's sweat and waste products.

Reduces Stress:

The heat from the saunas will cause the body to release endorphins along with other 'feel good' chemicals. These reduce feelings of stress on the mind and body. A lot of people feel rejuvenated and very calm once they have had a sauna or steam room experience, and are ready to tackle whatever is necessary for the remainder of the day.

Post-Workout Relaxation:

Post-exercise, your muscles are in desperate need of some relaxation to promote a quick and healthy recovery. When muscles become relaxed, the recovery process (which is crucial for muscle gain) is accelerated, and muscles can grow faster.

Can Aid in Weight Loss:

Regular visits to steam rooms or saunas can possibly aid in weight loss. It is well-known that saunas get rid of excess water weight. Although, it is important to note, this isn't in replace of a balanced diet with exercise, and instead, something you should use as an addition.

Unblock Sinuses:

The heat from a sauna or steam rooms will open and thin the mucous membranes. A lot of people come to notice their mucus has loosened and instantly breathe more comfortably, compared to when they first entered a steam room or sauna.

Keeping this in mind, saunas and steam rooms can be used to aid in ridding yourself of a cold too, as they can stop blocked and stuffy sinuses and aid breathing.

Promote Healthy Blood Flow:

The body's capillaries will become dilated when exposed to the heat of a sauna or a steam room. This allows blood to flow freely and efficiently around the body, and transporting vital oxygen to all areas of the body and mind helps this to occur.

Increases Flexibility:

Stretching stiff muscles before you enter a sauna or steam room will lead to the heat penetrating tired and stiff muscles. This makes them more fluid and looser, as well.

If you have access to a steam room or a sauna, then this is an excellent way to do all of the above. If you don't have access, you can soak in a bathtub. With the temperature higher than your body's for a 10-minute soak, make sure you DO NOT perspire for more than this 10 minutes, or you can lose too much nutrition from the nutrients which will be expelled in the liquid being eliminated from your pores, as mentioned earlier.

6

―――――――

NON-FAP

Professional athletes abstain from sexual activity before matches and they have been documented greatly and globally for doing so. But why is this? And what does this have to do with your hair, anyway?

The connection between sexual activity in men and hair loss has been noticed in both Taoist and Ayurveda (Indian) medical texts, for thousands of years. In a nutshell, it is maintained that excessive emission by men during intercourse (or otherwise, in masturbation), results in pattern hair loss for those genetically predisposed to this condition.

I personally, not only feel better overall, but my hair benefits from it greatly. I find my hair looks healthier and has a great sheen after abstaining for a week. To put it into perspective, and according to scientific research, when a man ejaculates he loses around a tablespoon of semen. The nutritional value of this amount of semen is equal to that of two pieces of New York steak, ten eggs, six oranges, and two lemons combined. That includes proteins, vitamins, minerals, amino acids; everything! It also creates great amounts of DHT, the enemy of hair, in high doses! So, imagine someone who; let's say, ejaculates 1-2 times a day, that's a lot of DHT, and a lot of nutrients taken away from their hair, because, at the end of the day, the organs receive the nutrients first. The the skin and hair get nutrients last, as a survival defensive mechanism. And so, if you are ejaculating all the time, then you're not getting very many nutrients to your hair at all.

The semen also contains a great deal of vital energy; therefore, an ejaculation also represents a great deal of lost energy in this regard. This is demonstrated by the exhaustion felt by the man after ejaculation. So, the conservation of sexual energy will not only aid the condition of the hair, but also the entire body. When adequate sexual energy has been conserved for an adequate length of time, a slow transformation of the body will commence. Balancing the energy within the entire body will automatically provide hair cells with adequate nourishment to grow hair with a beautiful, natural sheen, even in the most-seemingly hopeless cases. I highly recommend **"The Tao of Sexology"** by **Dr. Stephen T. Chang** if you want to learn more on this subject. But, the take away from this chapter is to abstain from ejaculating every day. Once to twice a week, at most, would be the recommendation. Test yourself; abstain for a full week and I bet you a million dollars (in Monopoly money) that you will feel like a million dollars, and your hair will significantly improve too.

7

NUTRITION

When trying to re-grow your hair and reverse baldness naturally, there are some foods you should minimize or avoid fully. In some instances, some food groups can actually trigger hair loss, so, reducing the amount of those can have a remarkable influence on your hairline.

On other occasions, it might not be one food, in particular. However, combinations of foods over long periods can have an effect. There are a few general rules when it comes to foods which are favorable to improving hair loss, while some specific foods should certainly be avoided.

Remember, vitamins and minerals we consume are vital to hair health, too. Ultimately, each constituent adds to the whole picture. Sometimes supplementation is needed because we don't get enough from foods. Eating organic is also vitally important, where possible. Your blood quality is extremely important, and its oxygenation is vitally important for whole body health as well as hair health.

Cutting out simple carbs, avoiding excess red meat consumption, refined sugars, dairy, and wheat is necessary. Replace these with complex carbs including brown rice, pasta, vegetables, white meat, seafood, soy, and beans.

The first universal rule is to avoid foods that might be causing delayed allergic reactions. These are comparable to instant allergic responses that peanuts or shellfish can often induce. However, these would occur over a period of weeks or days and are, therefore, more deceptive, but no less detrimental.

The primary reasons delayed allergic reactions aid in causing hair loss is due to increased immune responses which cause our bodies to attack hair follicles and cause inflammation in the scalp. This then restricts blood flow to the hair follicles.

The second general rule is due to acidic and alkaline foods. This is a broad subject, although, the general rule of thumb is to maximize the intake of alkaline foods and reduce acidic foods in your diet. Over time, this can considerably reduce the rate of hair fall and potentially aid in hair regrowth, too. Let's have a look at which foods can go toward causing hair loss, and should consequently be avoided as much as possible.

They include:

Dairy

Worst thing for your hair, ever! As well as being highly acid-forming once in our bodies, dairy can also cause delayed allergic reactions, and for both of these reasons, it ought to be avoided.

Commercially purchased dairy products are almost-always pasteurized, and this process of pasteurization essentially renders the naturally occurring enzymes useless or non-existent.

It is through this enzyme that humans are able to digest milk in the first place, and, without it, our bodies struggle to digest the dairy, making it bio-unavailable and of no use (nutritionally) to the body.

Dairy can also block the pores resulting in pasty skin. It also means epidermis plaque is more likely to build up on the scalp causing hair follicle shrinkage and thinning hair. For this reason, only try and consume unpasteurized dairy, or avoid it altogether. We get enough calcium from other foods, so, as long as your diet is whole food and nutritionally based, then you don't need dairy.

Carbonated Drinks

These produce high amounts of acid and are, in fact, the highest acid-forming beverage. Not only this; the quantity of sugar in them also causes blood sugar levels to spike which is followed by a crash.

Dr. Mercola researched links between excess blood sugars and male pattern baldness, and this is what he had to say about it. *"There is strong evidence that early male-pattern baldness could be a clinical marker of insulin resistance, a condition in which you lose your sensitivity to insulin, resulting in excess blood sugar."*

This specifies another overall rule: eat foods with a low glycemic index rating to help reduce the chance of spiking blood sugar levels. This has become a very significant concept for the reversal of hair loss and thinning hair. We must come to understand that male pattern baldness is an unusual problem; it is a modern 'ailment.'

The majority of processed foods all have ultra-high glycemic indexes, while natural (unprocessed, unpasteurized) foods contain a significantly lower glycemic index. This leads to the conclusion that there might be a link between processed foods, and the activation of the male pattern baldness genes.

Although this link between the two might appear unsubstantiated to some, there is further research which also came to a conclusion which was very similar to Dr. Mercola's. Alcohol consumption can also cause hair loss.

Rather than drinking carbonated or alcoholic drinks, stay hydrated with these instead:

1. Avoid pure tap water. Drink filtered, distilled or ionized water instead.
2. Drink fresh vegetable juices - not store bought, but naturally made.
3. Almond milk is exceptionally healthy, and also almond oil has been shown to stimulate hair growth in mice.
4. Herb and spice mixtures - anise, cloves, ginger, cinnamon, and lemongrass, plus many others.

Sugary Cereals

Sugary cereals and dairy cause blood sugar level spikes which are correlated with early stages of male pattern baldness. These foods rank very high on glycemic indices, so they unavoidably cause blood sugar spikes which we now see as something very conducive to early hair thinning, as I have already mentioned. It's no surprise that an ever-growing number of men suffer hair loss. And when you look at a usual westernized breakfast of pasteurized milk and sugar-filled cereals, it fits.

Processed cereals have a very high glycemic load as the majority of the natural fiber from plants is removed during their processing. If this remained, it would cause it to be digested and be absorbed more slowly by the body. When the natural fiber is removed, sugars go directly into the bloodstream causing significant spikes in blood sugar levels.

This fiber is also beneficial as it sweeps clean the colon of obstructed mucus and leftover feces. The fiber prevents it from being reabsorbed back into the body and causing the condition known as toxemia.

The solution is eating natural, unprocessed foods which contain high amounts of fiber. This is why it is recommended to follow a fast juice detox if you wish to beat your hair loss problem for the long-term.

Greasy & Fried Foods

These clog the arteries over time and also cause oily skin on the scalp. This, in many cases, leads to hair follicle reduction, restricted blood flow, and clogging of pores in the skin. Once the pores become clogged, DHT and other damaging hormones can become trapped and can trigger the hair loss mechanism to continue.

Side Note: Besides wanting your hair back, these types of foods should be avoided anyway, because they are the major causes of many of the debilitating diseases like diabetes, obesity, and heart disease, which seem to be the 'norm' these days. I know you're smart, so take care of your body; you only have one.

Foods That Will Help

A raw vegetable and fruit diet can help you reverse male pattern baldness. This type of diet really gets the blood and lymph systems flowing at their best.

I won't talk a huge amount about every food, because this would require its own book. And, at the end of the day, fresh fruit, vegetables, and whole foods are what the body (not only the hair) needs. I highly suggest you Google or buy books on nutrition and diet, and I believe that **The Tao of Balanced Diet** by **Dr. Stephen T Chang** is priceless in many ways. I will, however, speak about watermelon as it was something I did and still use for my hair loss, and I will tell you why.

Watermelon could be the best for hair stimulation as it contains high amounts of citrulline which dilates blood vessels. People use this as a way to improve erectile dysfunction because it acts like nature's form of Viagra. If it can help drive blood to your penis, there is a high chance it is improving blood flow to the top of your head, too.

Either by using a juicer or a blender, you can reap the benefits of watermelon; organic is best. You can also get similar results eating more of this fruit and by including other whole foods which are plant-based, like whole-grains, beans, nuts, and seeds.

Ginger - This common spice has been used for centuries in Ayurveda medicine in the treatment of hair. Ginger paste, when used on the hair, will reduce hair loss. Ginger is packed-full of essential vitamins and minerals, and the most important factor of all is it is an excellent stimulator of the blood.

Ginger can be an excellent remedy for hair regrowth, because it contains circulatory agents which aid in stimulating blood flow to the scalp. It also aids in activating the hair follicles and helps to grow new hair. Because ginger is a fantastic source of essential fatty acids, it prevents the thinning of the hair and eventually aids the prevention hair loss. It also has excellent anti-inflammatory properties by default. This can be combined straight into your watermelon juice, for use on affected areas of the scalp, via massage.

Remember, as mentioned earlier, vitamins and minerals we consume are vital to hair health, too. Ultimately, each constituent adds to the whole picture. Sometimes supplementation is needed because we don't get enough from foods. Eating organic is also vitally important, where possible. Your blood quality is extremely important, and its oxygenation is vitally important for whole body health as well as hair health.

Cutting out simple carbs, avoiding excess red meat consumption, refined sugars, dairy, and wheat is necessary. Replace these with complex carbs including brown rice, pasta, vegetables, white meat, seafood, soy, and beans.

Alright, so a quick note on other foods commonly used in the community. The garlic, castor oil and chili methods can be really useful. I personally have used them and saw results; HOWEVER, I discontinued them because, well, chili juice can seriously damage your eyes if it touches them by accident, and garlic absolutely smells and makes you smell like it for weeks, including your bed when you sleep. And, castor oil just makes your hair greasy and it's hard to wash out.

They are all great for hair loss because they are great penetrators. As we all know, rubbing garlic on your heel enables you to smell it on your palms within minutes. This is why they are so good, they penetrate the layers of the skin to get to the root of the follicle, to increase circulation and (in some cases) block DHT. But, I found something that was 100X more powerful without the smelly, greasy, and itchy consequences that come with the other methods. This will be discussed in a later chapter.

8

THE THYROID EXERCISE

HOW HAIR LOSS CAN BE CAUSED BY THYROID HORMONES

When your hormones get out of whack as a result of thyroid disease, your whole body can feel off-kilter. Your weight, your mood, and even your thinking can be affected, and you may have a host of other physical symptoms, too. Hair loss is a common side effect of thyroid disease, but it's not a permanent problem, as long as you get the treatment you need.

A person's hair follicles follow natural cycles of hair growth and inactive phases. At any particular time, the majority of a person's hair is growing, while a small percentage of it remains at the resting stage. When changes in an individual's body throw it off cycle, too much hair can rest at any one time, while not enough is in the growing stage. Actually, this results in the thinning of the hair, excessive hair loss, and ultimately, balding.

Numerous medical conditions cause hair loss, and thyroid illness is a commonplace culprit. Thyroid problems include both underactive thyroid (hypothyroidism) and an overactive thyroid (hyperthyroidism). As hair growth relies on the correct functioning of your thyroid, any abnormal levels of hormones produced by the thyroid gland will result in changes to an individual's hair. This could be in combination with many other adverse side effects, especially if it's left untreated.

When an individual has too much thyroid hormone being released, the hair on their head can become thin and fine all over the scalp. If there is not enough of this hormone, there might be hair loss, which can be anywhere on the body and not just on the scalp.

Oddly, if you take **levothyroxine** as a treatment for an underactive thyroid, this can contribute to some of your hair loss, along with other side effects. This only seems to be common during the first month of treatment, and more often in younger children, rather than adults. Looking at natural treatments is always recommended, because Big Pharma and western medicine doesn't always take into account the natural methodologies of health. See a professional if you need more advice, because thyroid issues can be detrimental if left untreated.

SOLUTION - THYROID MASSAGE

Merely by massaging the thyroid region can release energy into the thyroid to help it function on a more regular and cyclical level. Metabolism can be improved with this, and it enables the body to eradicate more poisons and toxins, too.

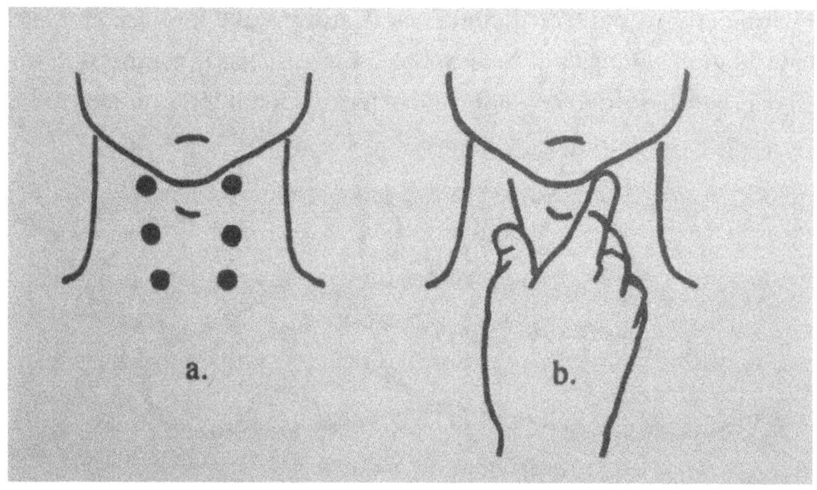

LOST HAIR & HOW NAIL RUBBING HELPS

This can confuse and excite a vast number of people in equal measure. How can rubbing nails help with your hair growth?

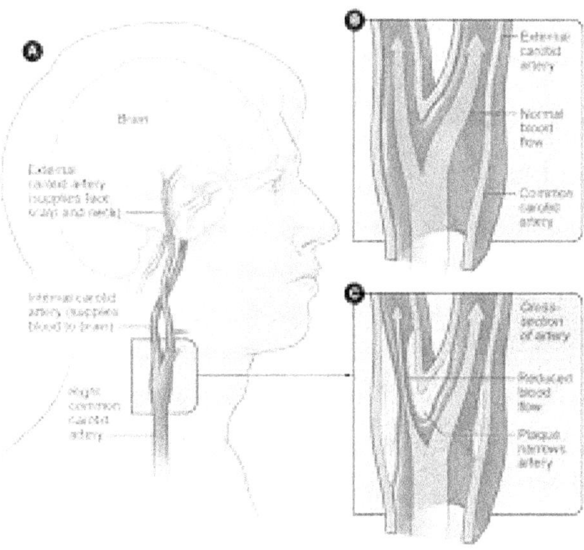

Here, the nail bed is made up of nerves which are connected to the scalp. With regular nail rubbing, blood flow and oxygen is stimulated to the scalp. Recurrent rubbing continually stimulates the scalp and helps rejuvenate hair follicles, while also enhancing your hair growth by controlling DHT (dihydrotestosterone). This can result in thicker and stronger hairs. Balayam (an ancient nail rubbing exercise) can even stop hairs graying, to some degree.

As an aside, it is shown to soothe headaches and help heal neurological disorders of the brain. Balayam to a high number of people appears a joke, at first. Through experience, it has been found that it's the most effective form of yoga for hairs, and the best natural remedy to help control falling hair and regain lost hairs through hair loss.

Balayam can be practiced by anybody, regardless of age or gender. In a good deal of cases, it works slowly but gently, and will produce the expected results after a long, consistent exercise of at least 6-7 months.

To produce expected results, nail rubbing exercises should be done daily for 10 minutes, split over four sessions of 2.5 minutes each(longer the better).

Warning: People with high blood pressure shouldn't practice Balayam as it could heighten their blood pressure.

Common factors for hair problems are:

1. Thyroid ailments

2. Hormonal imbalances
3. Smoking
4. Anemia
5. Heavy prescription medication
6. Hair dye with a high ammonia content
7. A vitamin B12 deficiency
8. A deficiency of protein
9. Old age and hereditary influences

Fingernail Rubbing:

Rubbing the left and right hand's fingernails with each hand can be a powerful practice to help to cure hair fall and to increase your hair growth.

Although straightforward, it is a very effective technique and a powerful hair-loss solution. Apart from being convenient, quick, and pleasant, this technique is highly relaxing and comes without cost.

The technique is tried and tested and definitely shows the desired results and it can be a potent amalgamated solution for all hair all problems.

How to Perform:

Hold your hands together and fold your fingers inward. Start by placing the fingernails of each hand against each other. Now with a regular swift motion, rub these against each other for 15 minutes, per session.

It is a straightforward technique and can be performed anywhere and at any time of day.

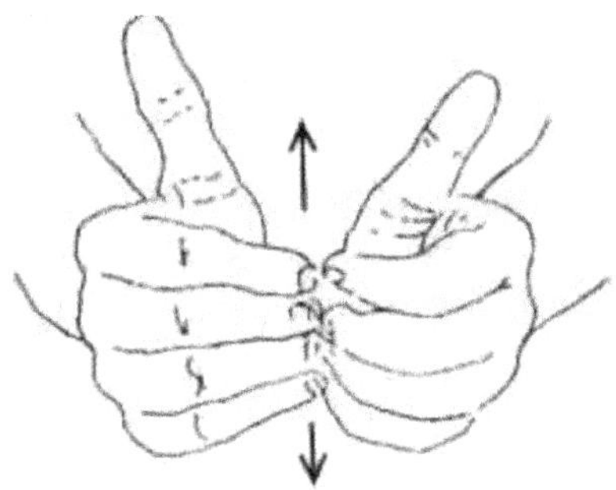

Fingernail Rubbing Benefits:

1. Aids in preventing hair loss.
2. Reverses the baldness issue.
3. Prevents the graying of hairs and restores natural color.
4. Typically it will take 3-6 months to see improvement from hair loss.
5. 6-9 months to see new hair growth.
6. Up to 12 months to see noticeable regrowth and considerable increases in hair volume.

The Theory behind it

Adult stem cells are homogenous cells which are found throughout the body after embryonic development. They can make duplicate copies of themselves for long periods of time, and reproduce via cell division to replenish any dying cells, while still regenerating any damaged tissues for self-renewal and self-healing.

Adult stem cells have the unique ability to heal themselves, and whenever tissue becomes damaged, adult stem cells are triggered to produce these new cells that can regenerate any damaged tissue, and revitalize the part of the body which was damaged.

These adult stem cells are most commonly found in the brain, spinal cord, blood vessels, and bone marrow, and also in other areas of the body, including the eyes.

Stem cells which are located in a hair follicle will, in fact, cause the hair growth. It is the rubbing of fingernails which stimulates the brain to send chemical signals toward these adult stem cells located in the damaged hair follicles.

The adult stem cells then rejuvenate and renew the base of the damaged hair follicles and with their ability of self-renewing, they then produce new hair follicles.

Now, with this fingernail rubbing technique, you can manipulate these adult stem cells which will become new hair follicles, and accelerate your hair growth by revitalizing any damaged follicles to reverse hair loss and baldness.

Reflexology:

Reflexology through stimulating certain parts of the body might directly affect other specific parts of the body too. Nerve endings which are just under your fingernails are directly connected to hair follicles, or your scalp. With the rubbing of your fingernails together you begin to increase blood circulation to your scalp.

Thus, the rubbing procedure (over time) increases blood flow to the scalp and helps with the strengthening of your hair follicles. This, in turn, reduces your hair fall and premature graying.

Precaution:

Be sure not to rub your thumbnails together as this might accelerate the growth of a beard, mustache, or other facial hairs. It can also increase hairs in the ears.

Avoid fingernail rubbing during pregnancy - rubbing nails could cause uterine contractions as well as elevating blood pressure.

Make sure to avoid it in some extreme surgical conditions; such as acute appendicitis, or angiography, or similar.

It should not be performed on problematic skin or nails if you have infected sores or lesions, or on brittle and diseased nails.

People who have a history of hypertension should avoid forceful rubbing of fingernails because it could elevate blood pressure.

Avoid any long, excessive, and vigorous rubbing as it might damage nails permanently.

Only rub the fingernails gently for 2.5 minutes per session, four times a day, for optimum results.

11

HAIR MASSAGING TECHNIQUE

THIS IS AN EXCELLENT EXERCISE FOR STIMULATING THE circulation in the scalp and for preventing hair from falling out, mostly because the hair follicles become nourished with added circulation.

Press your hands on the points of the head indicated in figure 1. Do not scratch these points; simply rub the skin back and forth without moving your hands from your head. Do so to massage the galea muscle to soften it up, as mentioned above.

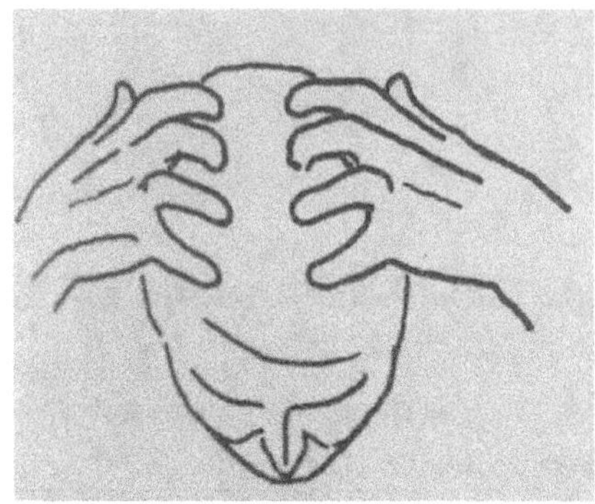

Here, the DHT will have made the galea tight and will be blocking the blood circulation, so you'll need to soften it up so that blood can reach the follicles.

After a few massages you will feel the scalp tension releasing and the galea becoming soft and allowing blood to reach the follicles again.

Practice this massage for about 1-2 minutes, three times a day. Morning, midday, and evening is crucial.

Here are some cheap and effective combs if you are interested, they are not vital, but are super-convenient, and I personally prefer to use them instead of my hands. This is mostly due to my hands getting sore after a while of massaging. And, if for any reason these items are no longer available, just Google any shampoo massage comb, there are a ton of them on the market.

Scalp Massage Comb 1

Scalp Massage Comb 2

Scalp Massage Comb 3

12

SECRET HAIR REGROWTH OIL

HAIR LOSS & FRONTAL REGROWTH

Here we explore the most amazing hair product for helping with hair loss: this is what trumps the garlic, chili, and castor oil ingredients. From all the compounds so far tried and tested, it is the topical emu oil which has consistently acquired the most encouraging feedback with respect to frontal hair regrowth. This is from many users seeing the instigation of vellous (fuzz) regrowth within just a few weeks.

It is well known that hair loss for the frontal regrowth is much harder to accomplish than any regrowth in the vertex, or crown regions.

This is particularly true of "FDA Approved" compounds of *Rogaine* and *Propecia*. Test data has shown these to be of practically no use in the stimulation of frontal hair regrowth.

Here we'll review the medical properties of topical emu oil, to give a further understanding of the numerous means by which it will support hair growth.

The emu (Dromaius Nova hollandiae) is a flightless bird which is part of a small group called ratites. This also includes the ostrich and the kiwi birds. The earliest emu oil research studies come from Australia, from where it continues to export emu oil to this day.

In the US, there is an ever-increasing network of research labs which are focused on emus and their "hard to believe" oil. This bird was originally imported as a peculiarity; a rare species which has many unique attributes. It has become the very source of an oil that when in its pharmaceutical grade form, is worth very close to $1,000 per gallon on the market. Most people tend to agree it's cheap at this price, considering the many health-promoting characteristics it offers.

Emu oil is rendered from hick pads of fat on the backs of the birds which are provided by nature as protection to the bird, mostly from the extreme temperatures in its Australian native homeland.

The fat is sensibly rendered to avert any formation of trans-fatty acids, and 100 pounds of the fat produces anywhere in the region from 50 to 90 pounds of pale, yellow-colored oil. This correctly-processed oil is made up of nearly 50% monounsaturated fatty-acids, while the remainder of it makes up its saturated and polyunsaturated fatty acid forms.

Studies performed in the Occupational Dermatology Laboratory located at the University of Texas Medical School in Houston have shown: 70% of the fatty acids in the emu fat are "unsaturated." These are the type of fatty acids that help protect the heart.

The second conclusion of this study is that oleic acid (which is a monounsaturated fatty acid) is the main component of emu oil. With that, and these fatty acids, it might well be the main reason for emu oil's amazing abilities to pass through the skin, and help with hair growth stimulation.

Emu oil is virtually 100% triglyceride, occurring naturally, which makes it an almost-entirely neutral lipid. Researchers feel it penetrates the human skin so readily and it contains a total absence of phospholipids.

Human skin is shown to be phospholipid deficient, and this means there is no phosphorus contained in the human skin. Anything put on the skin and scalp which contains phosphorus will not penetrate, as the skin is programmed to prevent such penetration from occurring.

Equally, anything like emu oil, which is phospholipid deficient (contains no phosphorus), will directly carry with it any medicinal benefits that are found within it. Even by itself without any added materials, emu oil includes some fantastic hair growth properties.

Emu Oil Properties

The most important property of emu oil is that it is highly penetrating. This ability to penetrate the stratum corneum layer of the skin has the potential for many new future uses.

Emu oil can be mixed with several medicinal lotions or cosmetic materials to carry them beneath this protective barrier, while also doing it cheaper than (and just as efficiently as) the costly liposomes and iontophoresis do.

At the present time, practitioners in Australia who specialize in hair growth use emu oil for these said penetrating abilities, because it gets into the scalp and really enhances the potency of topical medications.

In addition to this, it also helps the naturally-based medications to last longer. It is also anti-inflammatory, which could be (in part) the reason why it helps to stimulate hair growth. A group of four Australian inventors have segregated a yellow-colored component in the emu oil which appears to be one of the highest active ingredients, one which causes the oil's anti-inflammatory actions. They have since patented the substance which they isolated, and this patent along with further research could lead to a new raft of anti-inflammatory medicines in the future; which come with no adverse side effects. Coupled with this, they are found to be non-irritating, and continue to work while not being rejected by the body. One final note is this cream works out far less expensive than most, current, anti-inflammatory substances do.

Emu oil has also been shown to be used for the reduction of pain, swelling, and stiffness in joints, and can reduce bruising and muscle aches which is ideal for sport-related muscle strains.

Perhaps one of the most significant things is, it has been shown to impede tumor necrosis factor alpha (tnf-a). This is an inflammatory cytokine which has been shown to be actively involved in male pattern balding. Emu oil has also been proven to be a 5-alpha reductase inhibitor, targeting tissue when applied topically. It is this which is highly likely to contribute considerably to its hair regrowth properties.

Emu oil is an excellent emulsifier, and has good "blending ability." This means it can blend oils and water together, to then produce creams that have no oily residue on the skin or scalp.

The problem with most topical hair loss treatments is they don't penetrate the skin's barrier effectively. As we have previously seen, emu oil can penetrate this barrier efficiently, and do so without leaving an oily residue. This promises to be very good for its future uses in the cosmetics industry, as well as in future pharmaceutical uses.

Another significant property of emu oil is that it is bacteriostatic. Tests have shown that; while in a pure state, emu oil will not grow any bacterial organisms. Untainted, pharmaceutical-grade emu oil possesses a long shelf life for this very reason, as well as its low levels of polyunsaturated fats. These are subject to oxidation and eventual rancidity, however.

Emu oil has no potential for skin and scalp irritation and is shown to have no adverse side effects. This means that, even at full strength, emu oil has irritation levels which are so low they are comparable to putting water on the skin.

Emu oil is non-comedogenic which means it will not clog up pores and doesn't cause pimples when used. This is something which cannot be said for mineral oils (one of the most current and favorite carrier oils in cosmetics and rubbing oils) which will cause outbreaks of pimples or spots when used routinely.

Emu oil is a great moisturizer which adds to its already-fantastic protective ability and which promotes anti-aging of the skin. Researchers believe its unique combinations of saturated and unsaturated fatty acids could be the explanation for the high ability for the upper layers of the skin to retain water.

Like *viviscal* which is an expensive marine protein extract, emu oil can increase the thickness of human skin and the scalp, up to 2.5 times; this is thinner in male pattern baldness (MPB). This cures peri-follicular inflammation, which is an inflammation found around hair follicles which are affected by MPB.

The anti-aging factors of emu oil were proven in a study at the Boston University School of Medicine. A pharmaceutical grade emu oil was topically applied to debilitated mice for a two-week period in a double-blind study, while using corn oil as the control substance.

The processed emu oil produced an increase of 20% in DNA synthesis, which means growth activity in the skin of these mice showed a 20% increase. Also, the hair follicles were more robust, and skin thickness was also increased.

Dr. Michael Holick, MD, Ph.D., (who conducted all these tests) stated they had also discovered, *"Over 80% of the hair follicles that were asleep were awakened and started growing hair."* He explained hair follicles go through various stages of resting and growth. These follicles were awoken by the stimulation of them, which specifies it stimulates skin growth as well as hair.

Cautions:

As with any new product which blasts from obscurity to the mainstream, there are always cautions to consider and be made aware of. Emu oil was approved for use in July of 1992, by the FDA. However, it is still crucial you know that it is pure and processed correctly.

Both written evidence and research suggests it does all the things mentioned, although, as cautions, you must be aware there are some important questions and considerations to regard here.

Is the emu oil free from any contamination by hormones which might be generated if the bird is processed in an inhumane manner? And, is the oil free from any blood particles and meat scraps from inappropriate handling?

Was the oil being processed in a means that the trans-fatty acids have not been produced? This can happen when any oil is processed, and the heat is too high. These then cause numerous health-related issues as they are not now natural, and also not usable by the human body.

Is the emu oil product wholly free of solvents used in its processing? And is the company responsible for processing the oil willing to certify that this is so?

The better oils, whether from emus or vegetable oils, are made without any solvents being used during processing. Because this solvent method heats the oils to temperatures that (not viably) produce unwanted trans-fatty acids mentioned above. It can also leave non-edible solvent residues in the final products.

Has the finished oil been refined in a way by the use of a degummer (removes stickiness) in the product? And has a corrosive-based material like sodium hydroxide been used to remove phospholipids and other proteins? If these are used, they can cloud the oil.

Either of these steps is not appropriate; as the degummers will remove calcium, magnesium, iron, copper, chlorophyll, lecithin, and other phospholipids which are the contents required, enabling the emu oil to penetrate the skin's barriers.

The best emu oil purchased is low temperature processed, and highly stable and as close to its natural raw state as possible. Finding many good sources is possible. However, the earlier questions should be asked first. I personally get my emu oil from this site - http://www.hairloss-research.org/category/Categories-1 it is the cleanest emu oil in the market.

Dr. Holick Emu Studies and Results

Emu oil for hair regrowth in the mice was applied three times a day by Dr. Holick. Through personal experience, it was found fuzzy regrowth in the hairline occurred with a once a day application before bedtime, and with shampooing in the morning.

Dr. Michael Holick is a highly renowned endocrinologist who

specializes in the field of vitamin D and skin aging. He was employed as a Professor of Medicine at Boston University, and was also Editor-in-Chief of the journal called "Clinical Laboratory." Dr. Holick has, on many occasions, been awarded for outstanding personal contributions to the field of vitamin D research. His awards include the *Merit Award* from the National Institute of Health, and in 1998, he received **U.S. Pat. No.**5,744,128, for the topical use of emu oil in stimulating skin and scalp, and inducing hair growth.

Holick's findings regarding the hair growth stimulation and anti-aging skin effects of topically applied emu oil was detailed in an article named: *Study on Skin Enhancement and Hair Growth,* featured in *Drug and Cosmetic Industry Magazine.*

Excerpts are as follows:

"We found that there was about a 20% increase in the proliferative activity or the growth activity of the skin in the animals... And when we looked at the hair follicles, and the thickness of the skin, it showed that the hair follicles were much more robust and that the skin thickness was remarkably increased, suggesting... Also, we discovered in the same test that over 80% of hair follicles that had been asleep were woken up and began growing hair."

He also stated: *"A hair follicle goes through a cycle. It goes from a resting stage into an active growth period, and then it goes back to sleep again. We woke up all the hair follicles by stimulating them, and then we wanted to see if we could further stimulate these hair follicles by topically applying emu oil. We found that there was an enhancement in the growth activity of the hair follicles. So it gives us an excellent scientific indication that we were stimulating skin growth."*

Oil from free-range emus produces an expressively more pronounced anti-inflammatory ability, and eventually better hair growth due to the stimulating effects. This is due to plant lignans and anthocyanidins which are present in oils.

Dr. Holick obtained these effects with emu oil while applying it 3 times a day, in his study.

Another pilot study conducted in England showed hair growth stimulation effects on humans with Androgenetic Alopecia, when administered just once a day. 34 partakers took part in the study. Each was asked to apply the emu oil on their scalps on a daily basis. At the end of each month, the participants recorded the volume of hair on their heads by using a visual analog scale.

The found results were particularly encouraging, with many participants obtaining an average hair regrowth of 8.1% per month, and an average of 48.4% regrowth over the full six-month study period.

During this trial where the participants saw an average of 8.1% regrowth per month, the emu oil applications were made each day before bedtime, and a few drops were applied to the balding area, while being thoroughly massaged in. These results constantly fall in line with recurrent objective reports of emu oil stimulation regarding vellous hair growth (peach fuzz), within a few weeks of the initial application.

How Emu Oil can stimulate hair growth and prevent further loss.

• Inflammation incurred damage around follicles.

 Emu Oil is an anti-inflammatory that is more potent than corticos-teroids, but unlike corticosteroids, does not damage skin, blocks damage by inflammatory cytokines and free radicals.

• Miniturization of the hair follicles

Emu Oil increases follicle size and produces a thicker hair.

• The shortening of the Anagen (growth) Cycle seen in AGA, which gradually miniaturizes follicles.

Emu Oil increases follicle cell proliferation.

• Diminished micro-capillary perfusion (blood supply).

Emu Oil increases circulation and facilitates new capillary formation.

• DHT Accumulation, increased 5 alpha reductase Activity.

The fatty acids in Emu Oil are inhibitors of 5 alpha reductase and DHT production.

• Cutaneous fat layer decreases with advancing age.

Emu Oil increasese the cutaneous fat layer creating more robust , larger, better nourished hair follicles.

• Graying Hair

Emu Oil stimulates melanogenesis,(the production of melanin).

• Thinner Scalp

Emu Oil thickens dermis which is thinner in areas affected by AGA.

Emu Oil has been demonstrated to be the best penetrating of all commercially available topical oils and cosmetics, making it in addition to its singular effectiveness, an excellent trans-dermal carrier for other added hair growth ingredients.

The following photos were sent to us me by one of my friends that shows some readily visible evidence of hair regrowth in response to a treatment regime that is simply comprised of topical Emu Oil, scalp massage, and daily brushing with a Boar bristle brush, that reportedly stimulates skin repair mechanisms. What makes these photos especially revealing is the short, shaven down hair that makes the scalp completely visible. The top right and bottom left photos are the after shots.

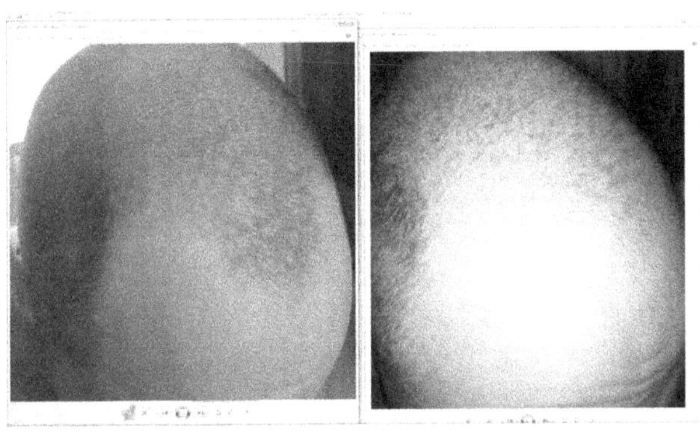

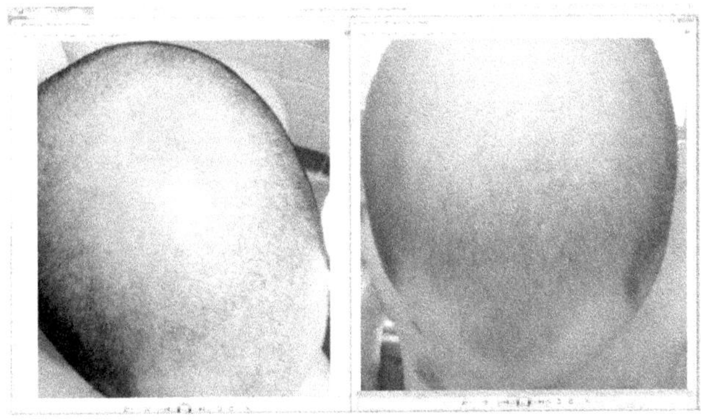

Although he was doing both scalp massage and Boar Bristle Brushing in addition to Emu Oil applications, theses photos generally reflect the feedback i consistently get regarding consistently applied, low temperature processed Emu Oil: A relatively rapid onset of vellous hair growth which becomes terminal over time.

Regrowth, as evidenced by these photos, can often be generated by even a modest regime. Faster and more thorough results can generally be obtained by more comprehensive treatment regimes, which incorporate systemic components that neutralize DHT, fibrosis, peri-follicular inflammation, and diminished Potassium Ion Channel Function, and additional topical components that stimulate hair growth factor in the blood vessel linings. Low temperature processed Emu Oil can either be used as sole treatment, or an adjunct to both Natural and Pharmaceutical Hair Loss treatment regimes.

13

DO USE HEADSTANDS OR INVERSION GRAVITY DEVICES

Not only does inversion make it easier for blood to run downhill toward the capillaries in the scalp, but the capillaries are opened further when baroreceptors in the neck and chest sense an increase in blood pressure to the head and act to reduce that pressure by dilating all the capillaries in the body (including those that service the hair follicles.

Invert yourself for 3 minutes per day morning and before bed at a 90-degree angle to increase the blood flow.

In general terms, as long as you build this up slowly and don't overdo the periods of inversion, a person should not encounter any unwanted side effects.

Nonetheless, if you find you have **any** of the following conditions it is recommended you entirely avoid using an inversion table:

- Vertigo
- Obesity
- Damaged or loose ankle and knee joints
- Pregnancy
- Heart or circulatory problems
- A hernia
- Low or high blood pressure, or recent strokes
- Detached retina, glaucoma, conjunctivitis
- Spinal injury, osteoporosis, ear infections

14

HAIR GROWTH SCHEDULE

So know that we know the many causes and solutions to hair loss, let's put them into practice and set up an easy to do schedule.

Morning:

1. So as soon as you wake up I want you to do the head massaging technique to soften the galea. Do this for about 1-2 minutes.

2.Next, do a handstand technique/inversion machine and let the blood really get down into your head, I personally use an inversion machine because I'm clumsy as hell... and I fall over all the time ;) 3 minutes.

3. Use the head massaging comb of your choice and really go over your head for a few minutes, do circular motions, and make sure you go over the frontal points as well. If you do not have a massage comb you can just use your fingers, and massage the whole head throughout. When you do this, you should feel a tingling feeling afterward; that's the blood circulating, this is good sign your doing the right thing.

4. If you purchased emu oil, place a few drops onto the affected areas of thinning, and areas of hair loss. Now rub in with fingers.

5. Do the Balayam technique (fingernail rubbing) it's easy! 2.5 minutes

6. Then lastly the thyroid massage for about 15-30 seconds.

All up; this should take no more than mere minutes to complete, and it's simple and easy!

Midday:

1.Again, like the morning, massage the galea, we want that nice and loose. Do for another 1-2 minutes.

2.After this, use the massage comb and go over your head, and, once again, really get into the areas of thinning and baldness.

3.If you bought the emu oil, apply the same as the morning method.

4.Do the Balayam fingernail rubbing technique.

5.Do the thyroid massage.

Before Bed:

Do everything you did in the morning, for the same amount of time and in the same order.

Galea head massage

Headstand or inversion machine

Massage scalp with hands or comb

Emu oil, if purchased

Balayam fingernail rubbing technique

Thyroid massage

I'd really like to make this clear; you do not need to buy anything for this to work. But, the hair-massage combs, the emu oil, inversion machine, and/or making your DHT blocking shampoos are definitely immensely helpful. However, you will grow your hair without them, and you can still do handstands without an inversion machine, and massage with your fingers. The higher the frequency you do these exercises, the better results you will get. So, do fingernail rubbing 4-5 times a day, thyroid exercise an extra time during the day, and so on. Making sure you have read all the cautions regarding these, first and foremost. But... if you want results fastest, make sure to get at least the emu oil, that's my damn best secret, ever!

Another thing that is the most important factor in this whole scenario is patience. Do not be discouraged if you don't see instant results, patience and persistence is a must with this. Remember, hair takes time to grow, they reckon a month per inch, so be vigilant, at the end of the day the schedule is quick and easy to do and doesn't require you to buy anything. If you can't do them daily for a month then (to be honest) you don't deserve hair, and I want you to enjoy having a shiny head!! Don't you? Great. Now you know what do!

15

HAIR SHAMPOOS

USE DHT BLOCKER SHAMPOOS FOR EFFICACY

When it comes to treating hair loss and regrowing healthy, strong hair, there is no "quick fix." These shampoos (while being beneficial) should purely be just another tool in your arsenal when you are faced with fighting male pattern baldness. And, to be honest with you, I refrained from using any shampoos at all; natural or chemical, in my hair loss journey. I simply used water and a boar bristle brush. So, while this chapter is dedicated to natural shampoos, it's not 100% necessary, but I just like giving people the options because it can be very beneficial.

Bear in mind that these shampoos will aim to block DHT. However, they won't reduce any of the sensitivity of your hair follicles toward DHT. This is the fundamental factual cause of hair loss in men with androgenetic alopecia. It should also be the ultimate goal for all those who are looking to regrow their hair.

When you are using these shampoos, it is consistency and patience which are vital. You shouldn't expect to see any results overnight, and you might have to experiment quite a bit with the many different shampoos and varying formulas to get the results you desire.

Don't forget, shampoo is merely a simple combination of a good cleansing agent, plus an essential oil and carrier oil, so it is possible that anyone can start making their own DIY hair-restoring shampoo.

Scalp Preparation

During our everyday lives, we will come into contact with many pollutants, chemicals, and other external elements which contribute to scalp buildup. We find, with this buildup, it blocks the hair follicles and varies the natural pH balance. This makes the scalp an unlikely place for continual hair growth.

This buildup can additionally make it more difficult for shampoos to even make it to the hair follicles. This is a requirement, especially if you accurately want to block DHT, while also minimizing the impact it will have on your hair.

So, before using any one of the all-natural shampoos, we need to use a homemade scalp exfoliate. It only takes a few ingredients to get started, and the results are a clean and restored scalp.

Ingredients:

- 1/2 a teaspoon of Himalayan or sea salt
- 1 teaspoon of powdered, activated charcoal

- 4 inches of ginger
- 1 whole cucumber
- 1 lemon, for juice
- A juicing machine - can use a blender and muslin cloth

Directions:

- First, juice the ginger and the cucumber then combine the juices in a container. If you are using a blender, combine both ingredients and blend up the mixture with the lemon juice.
- Drain the blended mix with the help of muslin cloth and keep the juice.
- Take 100 mL of the cucumber and ginger juice mixture, and add the salt and the powdered activated charcoal.
- If you used a juicer, make sure to add the lemon juice from one whole lemon.
- Mix the combination thoroughly.
- To apply the homemade mixture, gently massage into the areas of the scalp where you would like your hair to regrow.
- The lemon and ginger take some time before they begin breaking up any buildup, so, let it sit for 5-10 minutes.
- Rinse with warm (not hot) water.

It might require a few sessions before all of the plaque has been entirely removed. To help make it easier, you can lightly brush away any resulting flakes using a hairbrush.

DHT Blocker Shampoos

Now that your scalp has been prepared, it's time to take a look at the three shampoos below which will block DHT and combat hair loss caused by the miniaturization process.

3-Ingredient DHT Blocker Shampoo: Ingredients:

- 1/2 cup of liquid castile soap
- 5-10 drops of liquid nettle leaf extract
- 10 drops of jojoba oil

Directions:

- First steps require the preparation of the liquid nettle leaf extract.
- Finely chop four teaspoons of fresh stinging nettle, and set aside.
- Wear rubber gloves while doing. Fresh nettles can cause a mildly painful skin reaction when they sting.
- Fresh is always the best. Nonetheless, you can still make it with dry.
- Boil four cups of water, remove from the heat and add the chopped nettles into the water.
- Steep for a minimum of 20 minutes. Keep the pot covered the entire time.
- You might have to steep the nettles for longer to produce stronger extracts.
- Pour the resulting liquid through a small strainer or muslin cloth into another container. This you'll use to store your shampoo.
- Next, mix the liquid castile soap along with the jojoba oil to the container of nettle juice, and then mix well.
- To use, pour over wet hair and massage into the scalp for around 2-3 minutes.
- Rinse thoroughly with warm water.

Express Benefits:

The liquid castile soap is your cleansing agent in this homemade shampoo mixture, and it will gently help to wash away sebum buildup on the scalp. This could be from previous hair care products or any other chemicals which your scalp has previously retained. Jojoba oil is potent oil which absorbs deep into the layers of skin while still bringing infused ingredients with it.

Lastly, nettle leaf is a well-known DHT blocker. This can be when taken internally or applied externally. This powerful plant delivers a powerful anti-inflammatory punch and is an indispensable ingredient for anyone who is looking to decrease any scalp inflammation and irritation.

DHT Blocker Saw Palmetto Shampoo

Ingredients:

- 1 cup of warm water
- 1 tablespoon of baking soda
- 1 tablespoon of apple cider vinegar
- 5 drops of citrus essential oil
- 1 capsule of saw palmetto gel
- 2-3 teaspoons of olive oil

Directions:

- Mix the water, baking soda, vinegar, and olive oil.
- The baking soda and vinegar will react when combined, so be sure to use a non-airtight container.
- With the tip of a sharp knife, pierce the end of the saw palmetto capsule. Squeeze the gel directly into the above mixture and combine well, by stirring.

Express Benefits:

Both the baking soda and apple cider vinegar (when combined) make a gentle and powerful cleansing agent. This they do, without stripping away any of your scalp's essential oils. It thoroughly dissolves and washes away any excess oils and scalp buildup.

Citrus is an excellent antioxidant and is well-known to scavenge and neutralize the free radicals on (and in) the scalp.

Saw palmetto is the foremost DHT blocking ingredient. Studies show that any shampoos which contain saw palmetto improve hair growth by 35%, both regarding mass as well as volume.

Olive oil is a great carrier oil in this homemade shampoo recipe. However, it also hydrates and protects hair from breaking, without clogging any of the pores.

DHT Blocker Shampoo with Reishi and Green Tea

Ingredients:

- 1/2 a cup of liquid castile soap
- 1/3 of a cup of aloe vera gel
- 1/2 a cup of green tea
- 10 drops of vanilla essential oil
- 1 cup of reishi mushrooms

Directions:

- Add the reishi mushrooms to a pot of boiling water, then remove from the heat and set aside to cool.
- Once cooled, remove the reishi mushrooms and discard.

- Mix one cup of the reishi extract with the remaining ingredients, stirring to thoroughly combine.
- Apply the mixture to wet hair and massage into the scalp for 2-3 minutes.
- You can let the shampoo sit for 5 minutes.
- Rinse thoroughly with lukewarm water.

Express Benefits:

The above combination of healthy ingredients can cleanse, nourish, and moisturize the scalp, while at the same time decreasing DHT levels and inflammation.

The aloe vera gel performs as an alkalizer and brings the pH of the scalp back into a natural balance. It also soothes irritation and any itchiness.

The compounds found in the green tea, such as polyphenols and flavonoids, will helpfully contribute to the hair's growing properties. It is also known to be a blocker of DHT.

Vanilla essential oil works by stimulating new hair growth, and the reishi mushroom extract inhibits 5-alpha reductase, which is the initial cause of DHT production.

Let's reiterate some things, a small revision–

Causes:

- testosterone balance with regard to hair loss
- Role of blood and circulation in the scalp (galea)
- The role of low thyroid hormones with regard to hair loss
- Dietary changes to improve hormone health and help regrow hair
- How to avoid chemicals that may disrupt or increase hormones and play a role in hair loss

The Regrowth Program

Practice the hair schedule daily! Yes, 3 times, as a minimum.

1. Dietary changes such as avoiding grain products, refined

    sugar, and foods that may potentially disrupt thyroid activity (diary especially!)

2. Do the massage schedules everyday, no days off!

3. Avoiding shampoo - using only water and scrubbing to clean hair (both to reduce sebum production and to avoid the potentially hormone-disrupting chemicals).

4. Try and get yourself into a sauna or a steam room 1-2 times a week.

5. Try the 10-day no-fap test - you will feel amazing! And your hair will too.

6. Persistence! Keep at it; don't stop! Your hair will come back if you don't stop! Keep going; it's super-easy!

All in all, the information above is easy to do, and it's quick and makes sense. It is also based on scientific proof and my own personal hair regrowth story. It could cost you a bit if you went all out, or it can cost you nothing, and it will just take slightly longer to do. Also you may reduce the exercises to every second or third day once you have your hair back.

But, whatever the case, your hair will come back with patience as the major key. All you need is the blood to the roots of the follicles, which is so simple; it's not even funny. The massaging will break up the DHT as mentioned, so all is covered.

One final thought, you might have: it is often assumed that hair that is lost in pattern balding somehow "dies" after a certain period of time, and is therefore gone for good, rendered incapable of regeneration. This assumption is also erroneously reinforced by certain doctors, and other hair specialists. The following case study was published in a reputable peer reviewed journal, along with numerous anecdotal accounts I have received over the last couple years, and they convincingly refute this assumption.

This particular study gives an account of a 73-year-old man who had been completely bald since 28, regrowing a full head of hair at age 73 (45 years of slick baldness) after 6 years on oral spironolactone, effectively shattering the assumption of "dead" hair follicles. This 73-year-old white male had been bald since the age of 28. He developed nonA-nonB-induced liver cirrhosis and had been treated with spironolactone for the last 6 years. For the last 3 months, his hair had started to regrow over the scalp.

The fact is, that hair follicles technically never "die," in fact, they miniaturize to the point that they are no longer visible over time, resulting in a slick bald appearance. Once a hair follicle miniaturizes to this point, it does become extremely resistant to treatment and regeneration. Researchers at L'Oreal and other academic institutions identified the culprit behind this resistance to regeneration, as a progressive and longstanding fibrosis (chronic inflammation induced collagen hardening) that occurs in Androgenetic Alopecia. Perifollicular Fibrosis and the resultant miniaturization occur in response to inflammation and DHT, making it almost impossible to regrow hair in completely bald areas, in the short term. However, as fibrosis is gradually reversed, regrowth of hair is possible, and as this study shows, it is possible in the long-term not matter what age you are.

So with that final note, LET'S GET TO IT!!